Copyright © 2017 Alena Knezevic
All rights reserved.
ISBN-13: 978-1979761758

Bright Smile
Dental Coloring Book

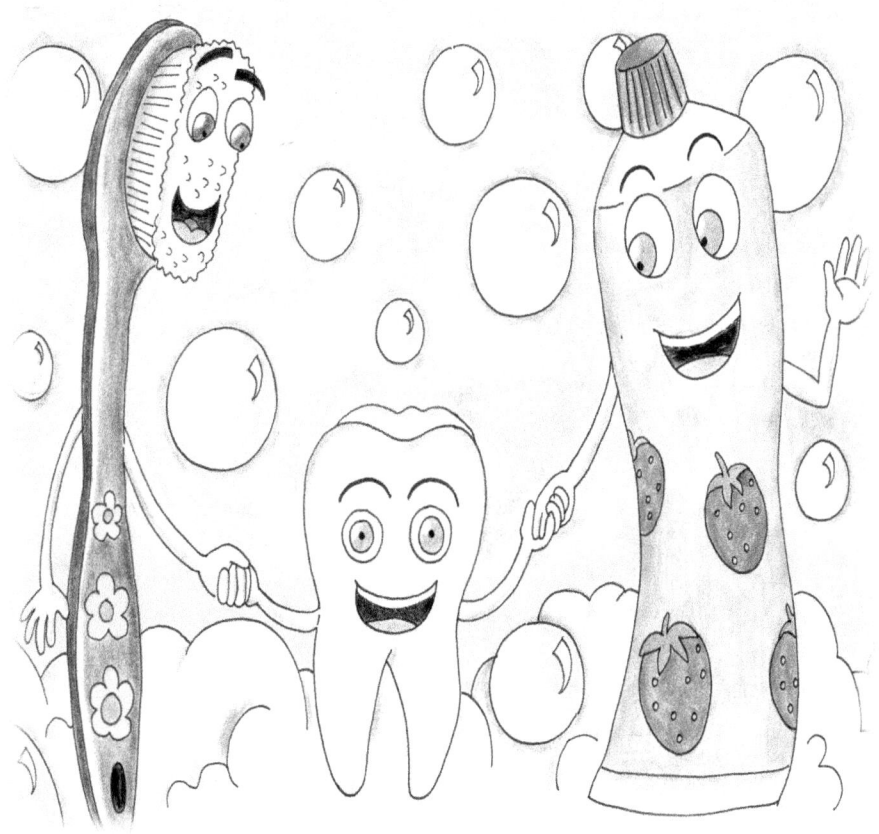

Alena Knezevic DMD, MS, PhD

Illustrated By Rina Risnawati

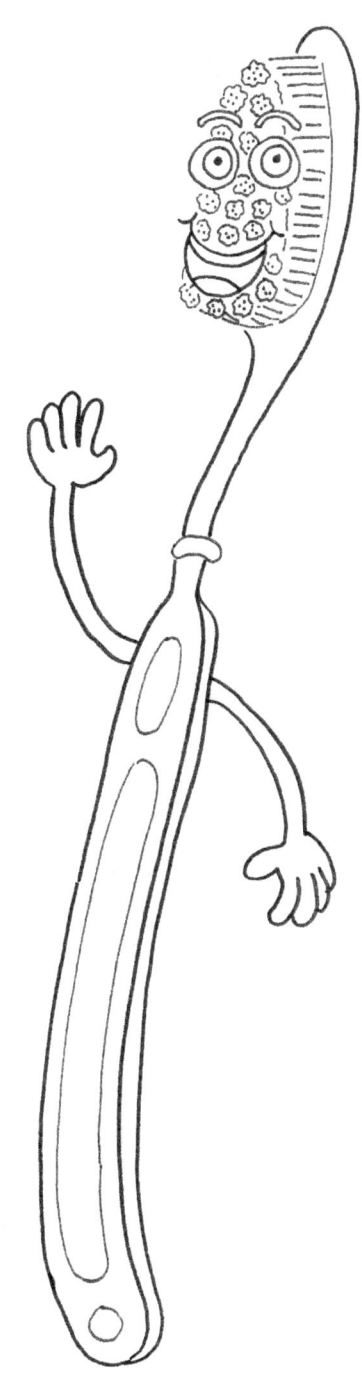

Hello, my name is brush – Toothbrush!

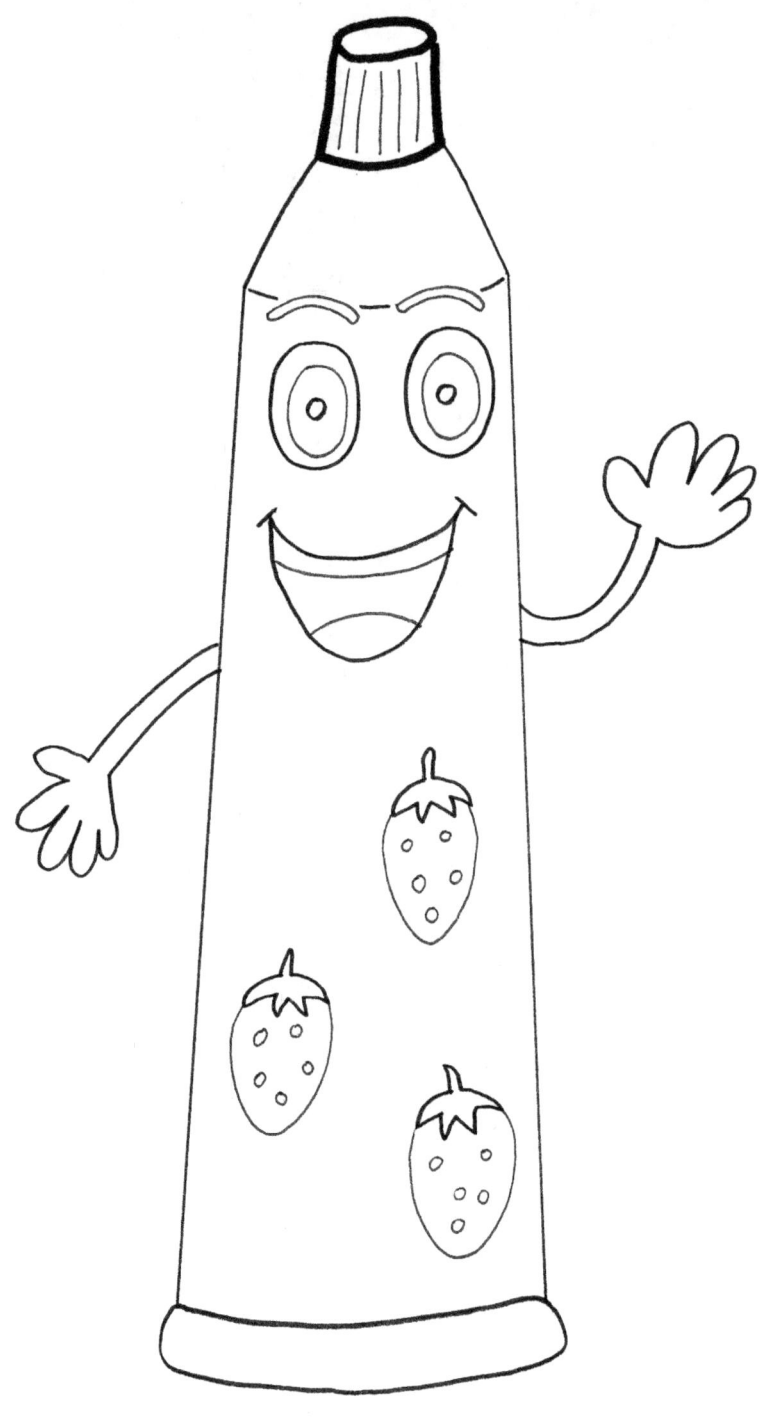

And my name is paste - Toothpaste!

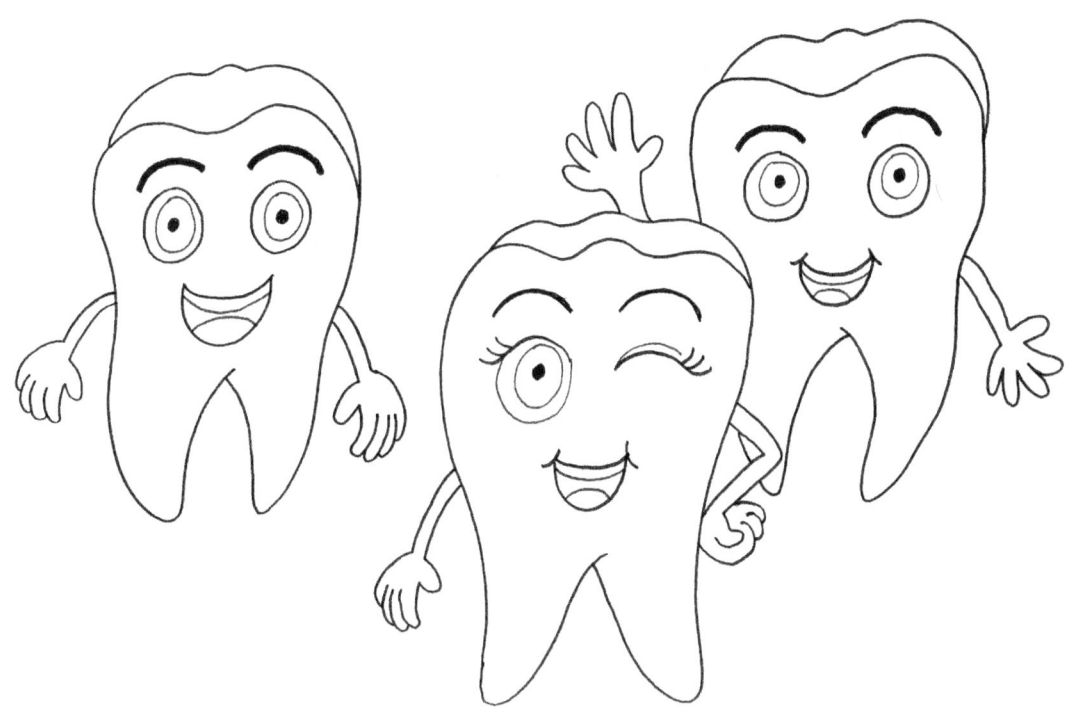

And do you know who we are?
We are your teeth!

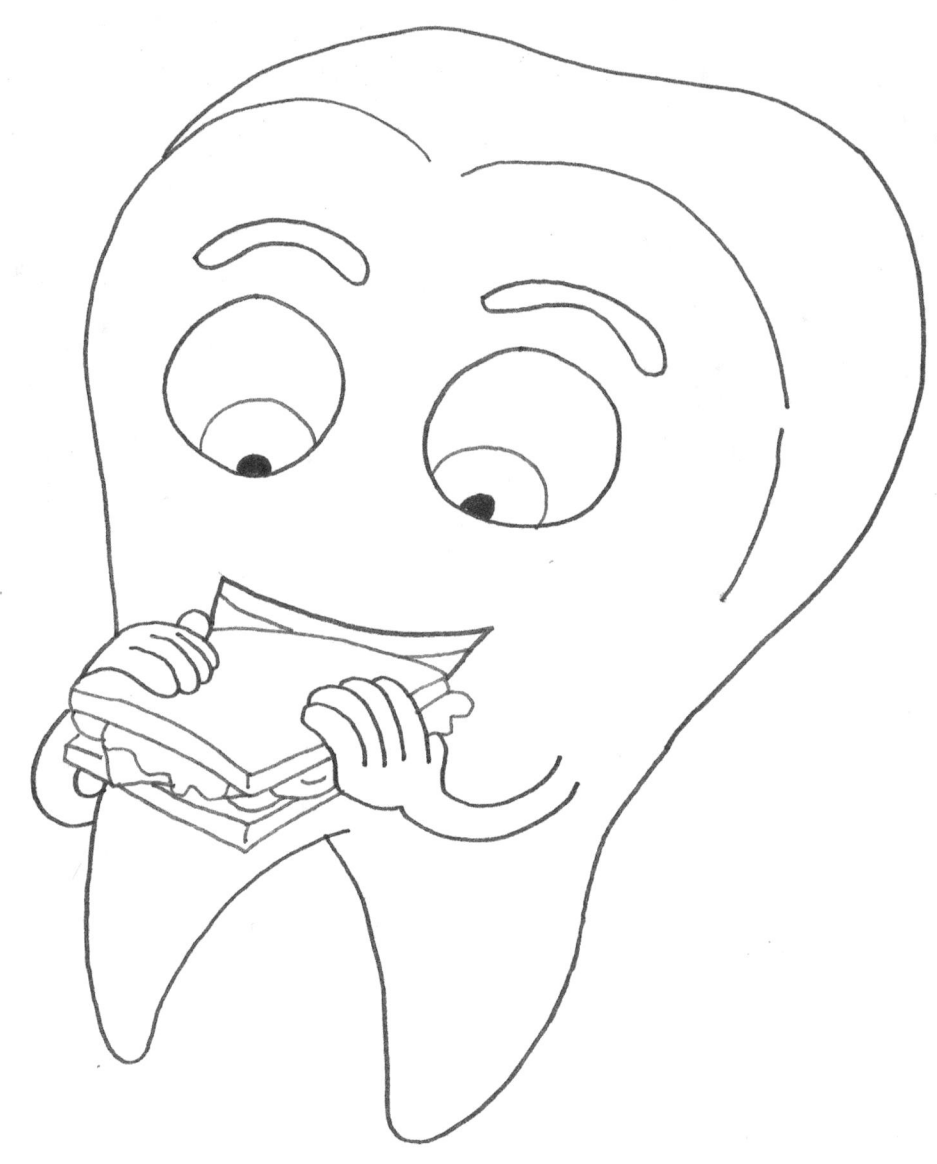

The teeth that help you to chew food ...

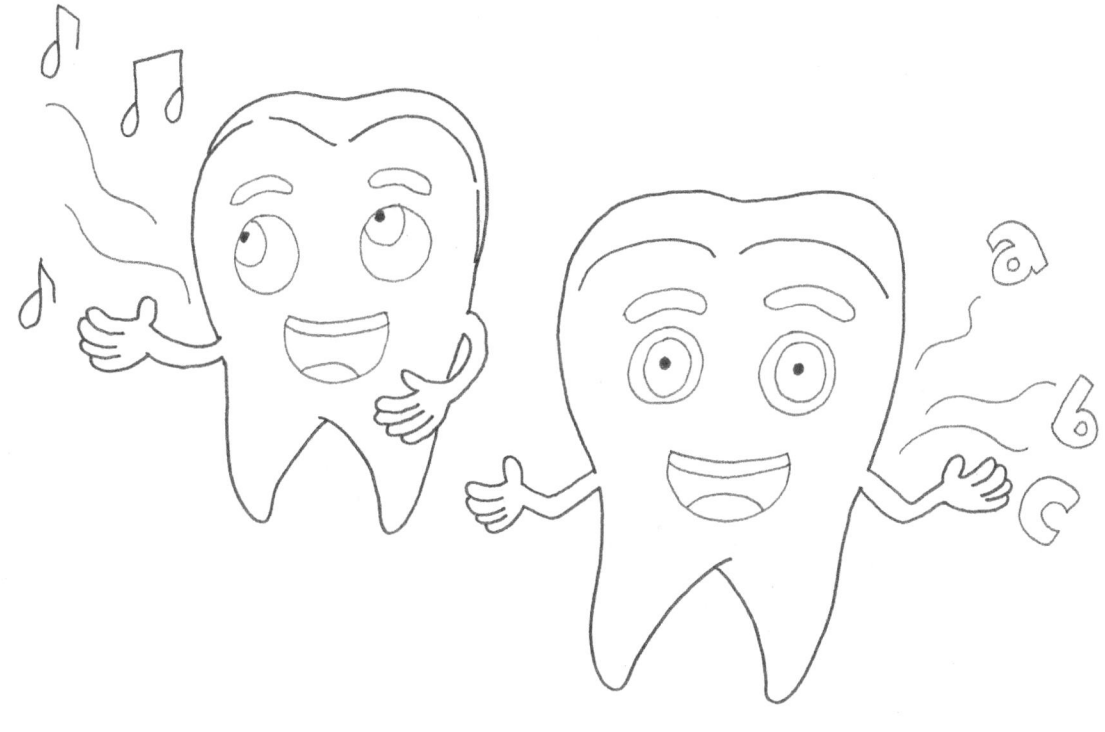

... make sounds while you speak and make you beautiful when you smile!

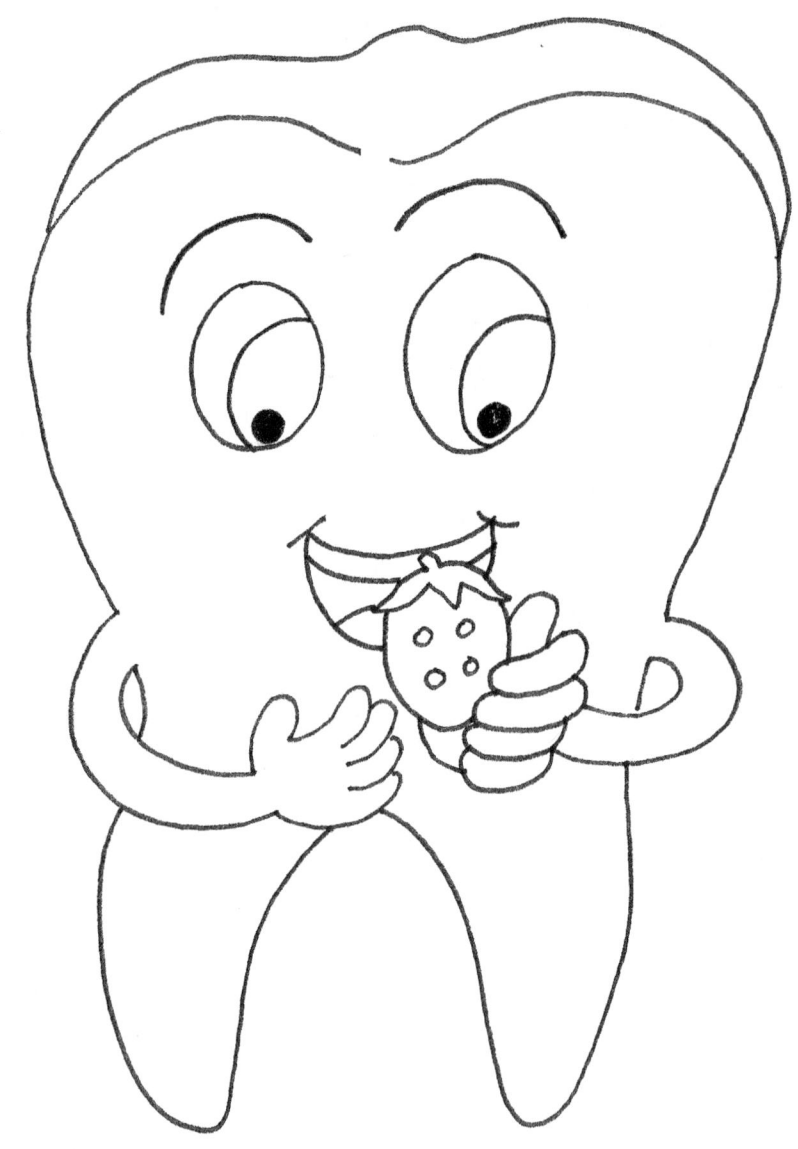

You have to keep us clean and feed us and yourself with healthy food.

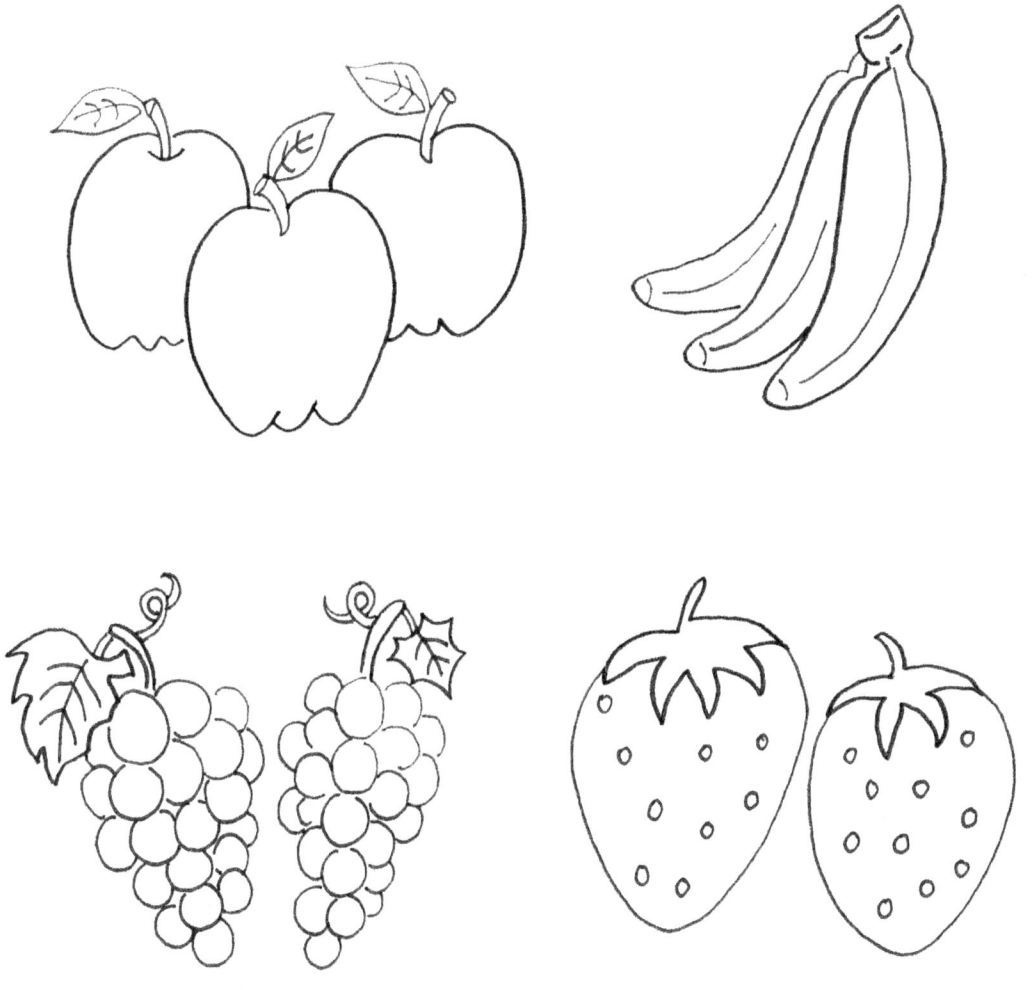

Eat a lot of fruit!

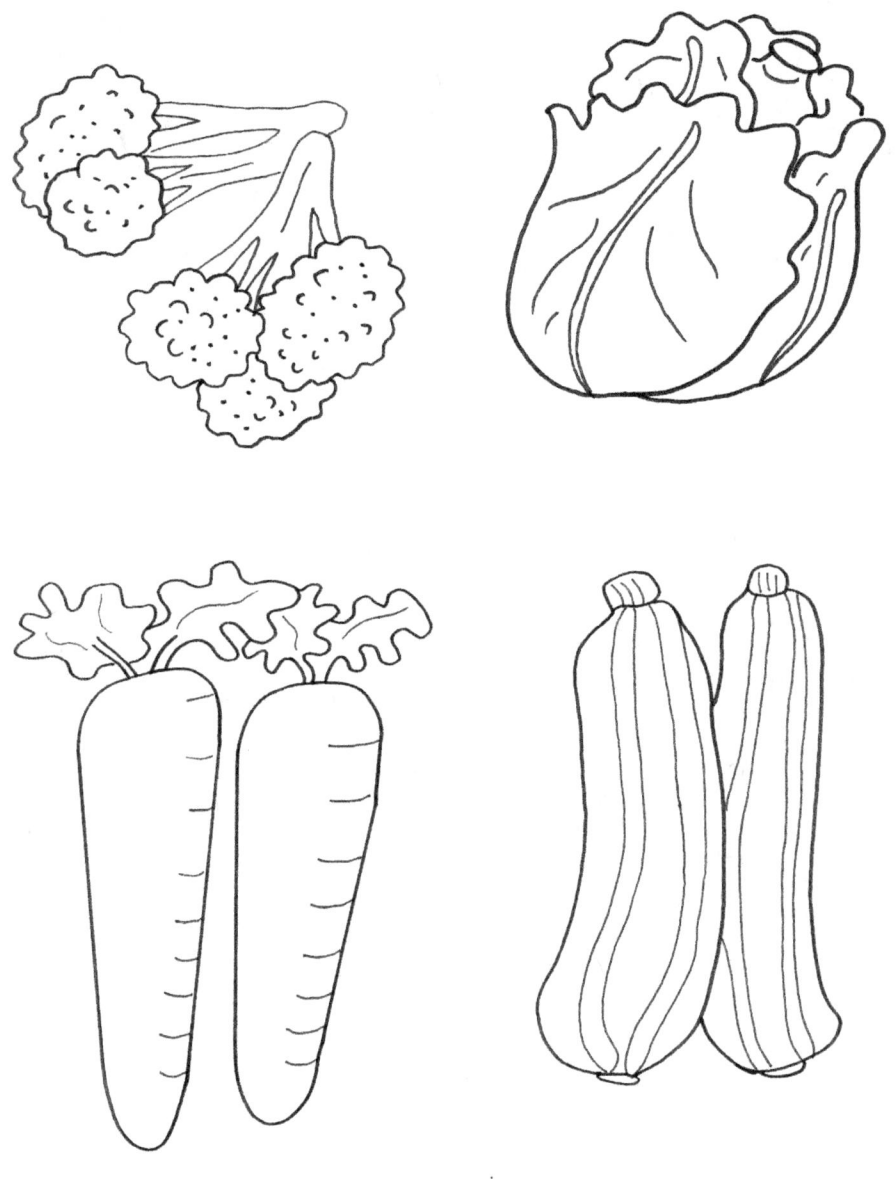

Eat a lot of vegetables!

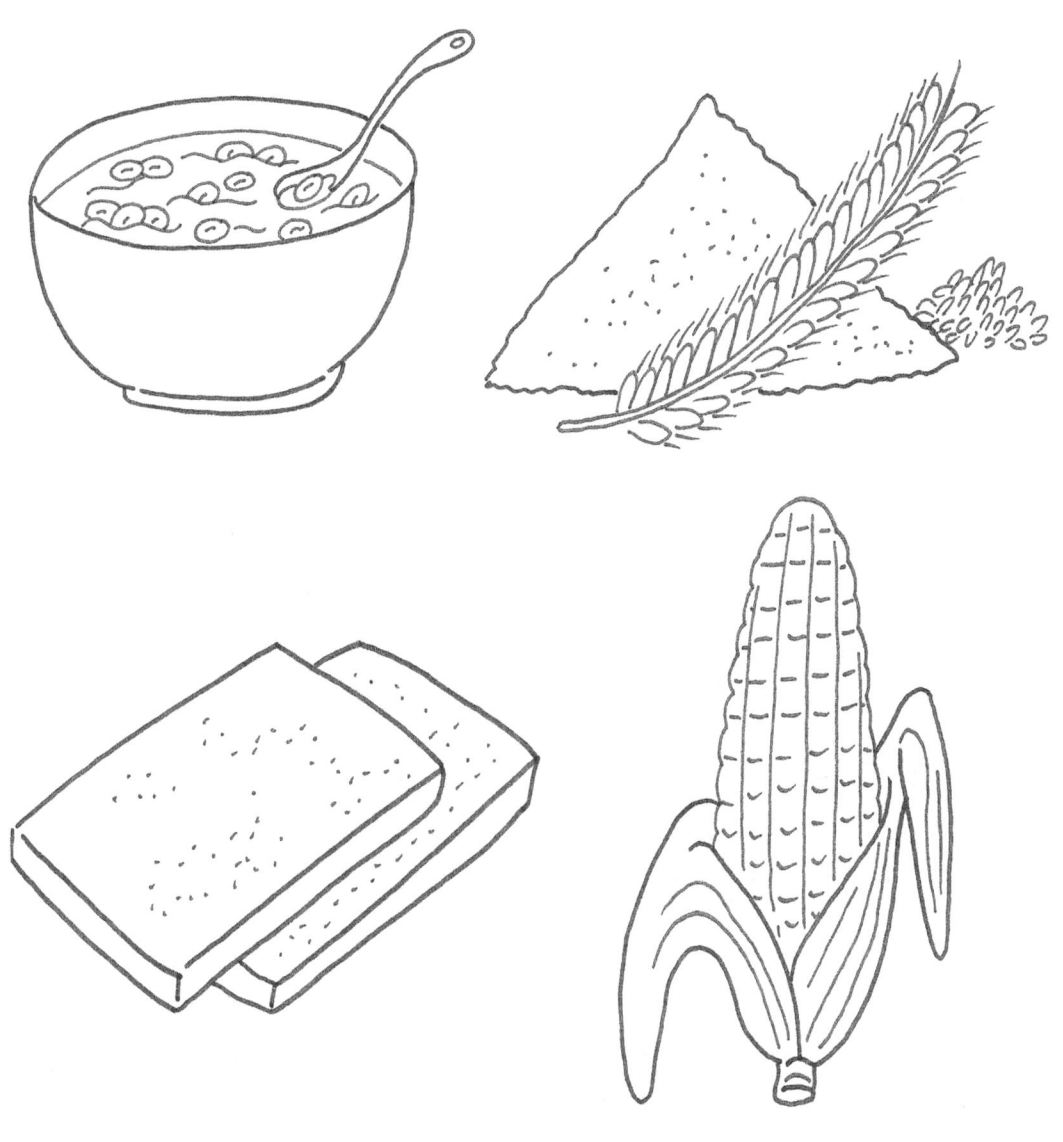

Eat a lot of whole grains.

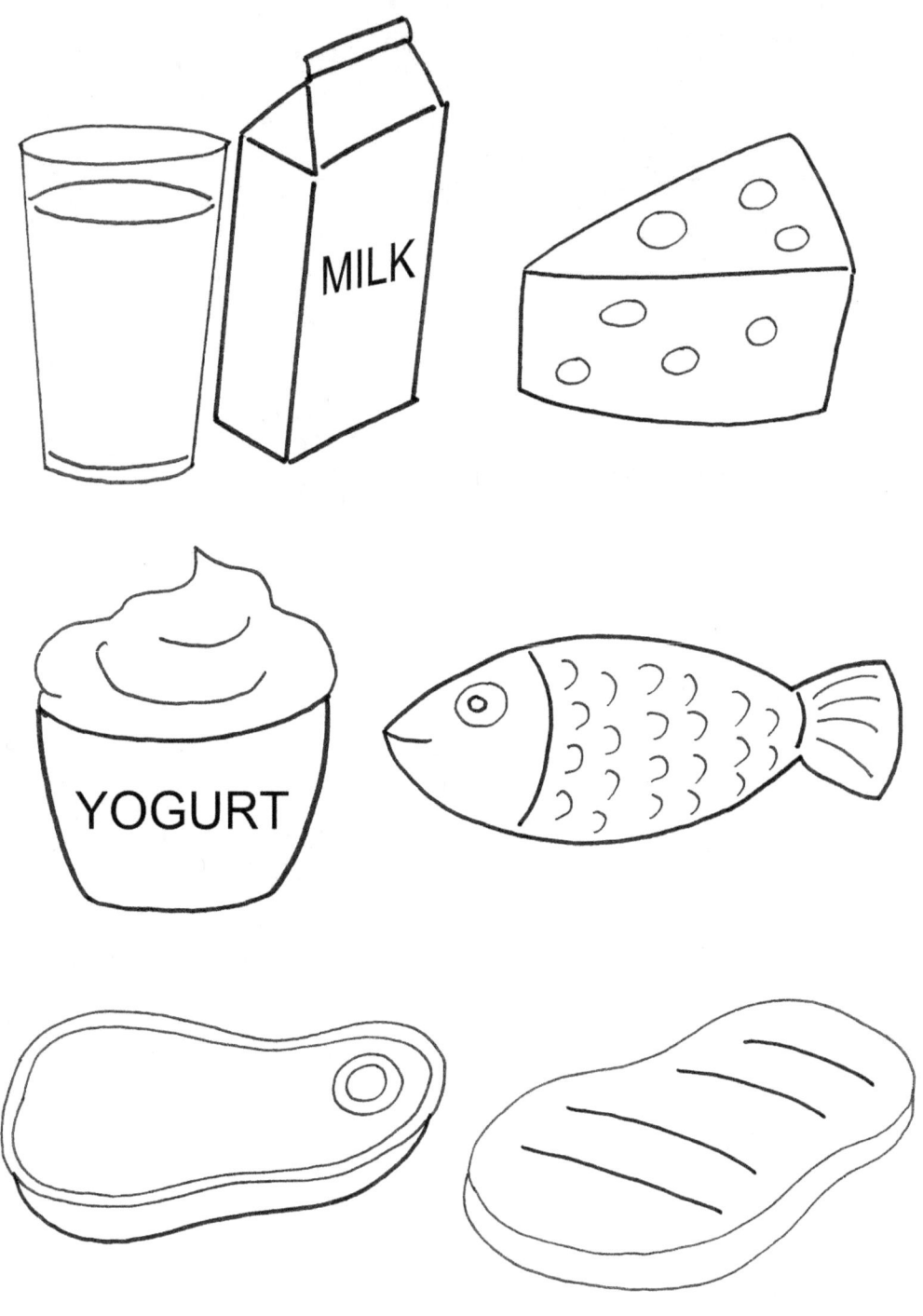

Eat a lot of dairy products and proteins.

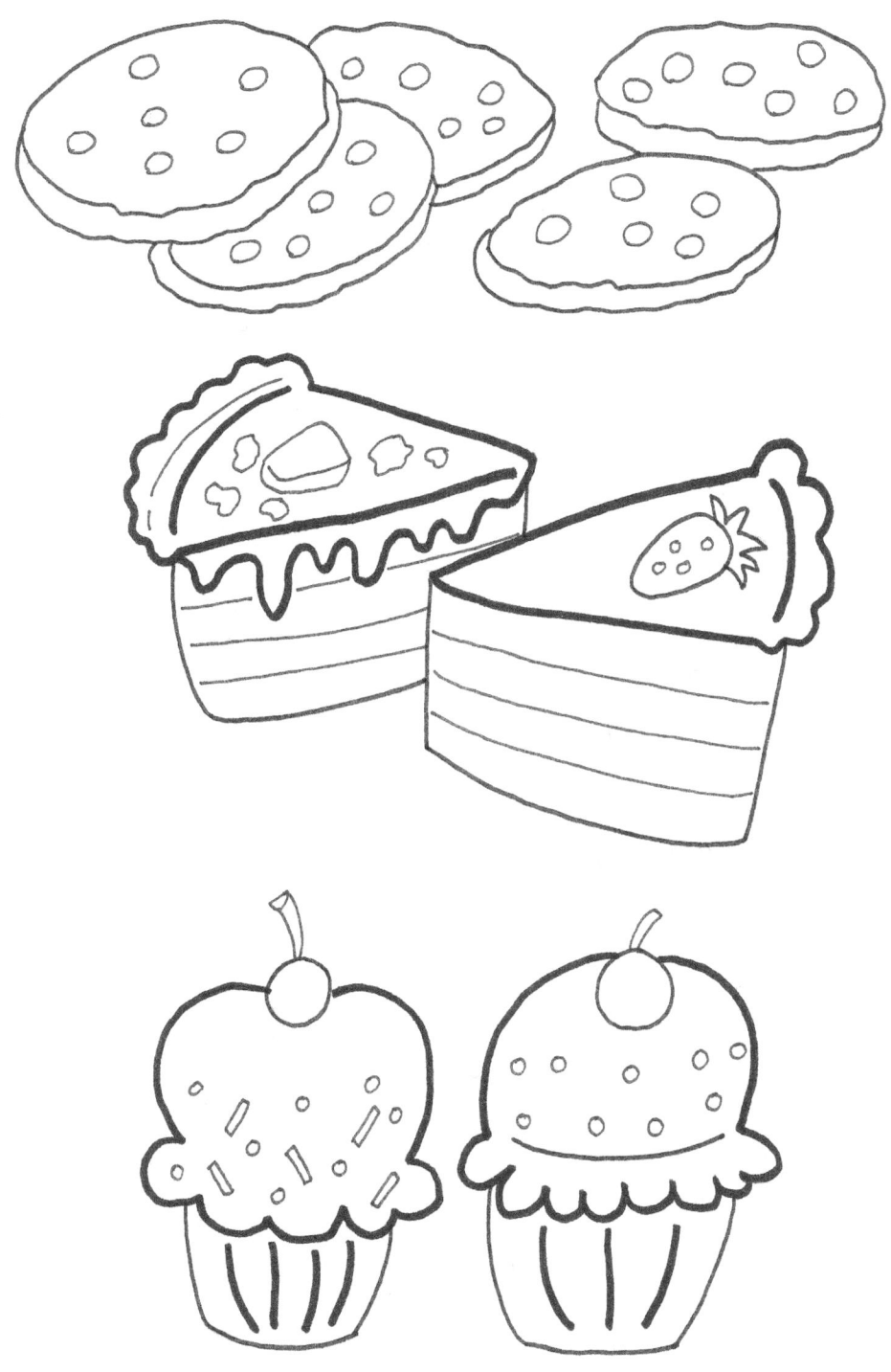

But avoid eating cookies.

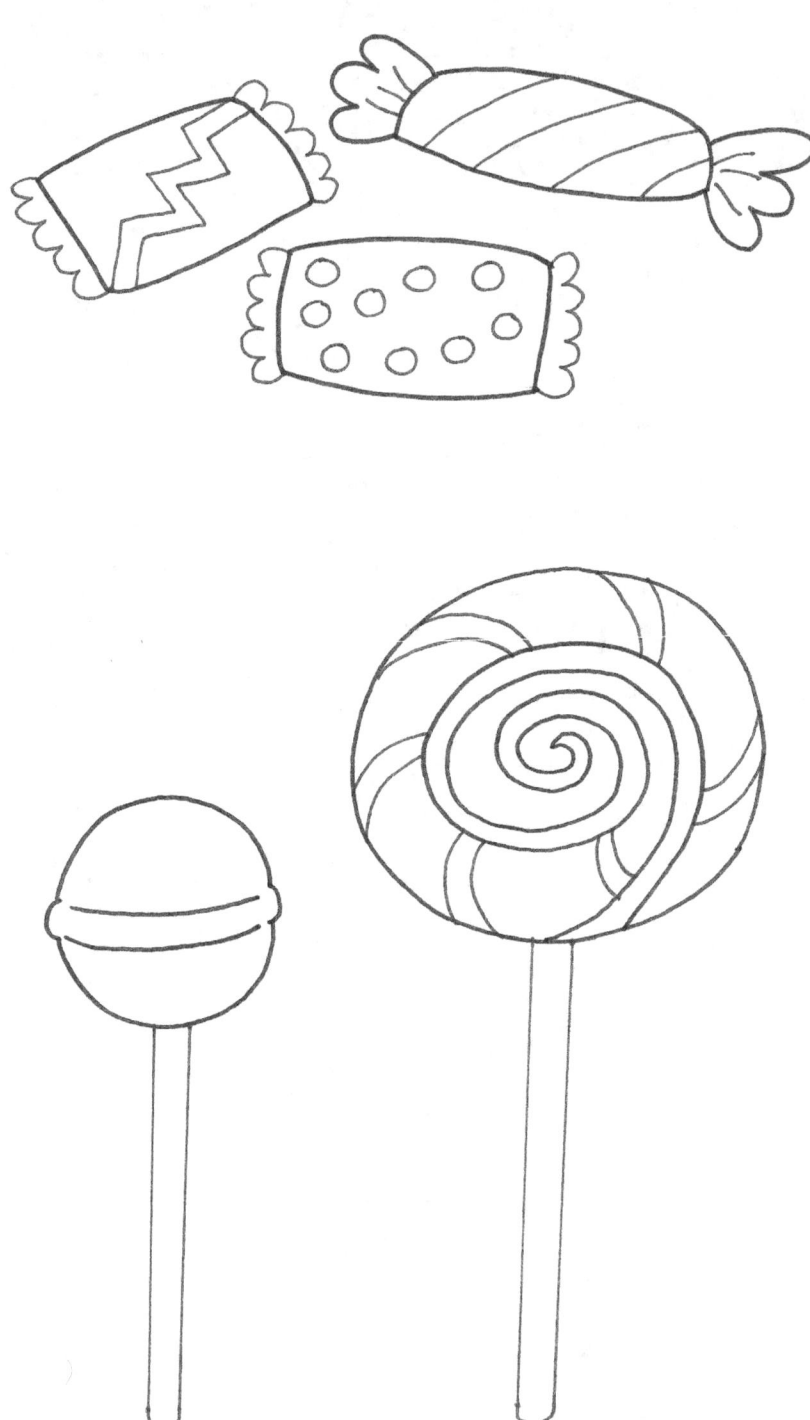

Avoid eating candy!

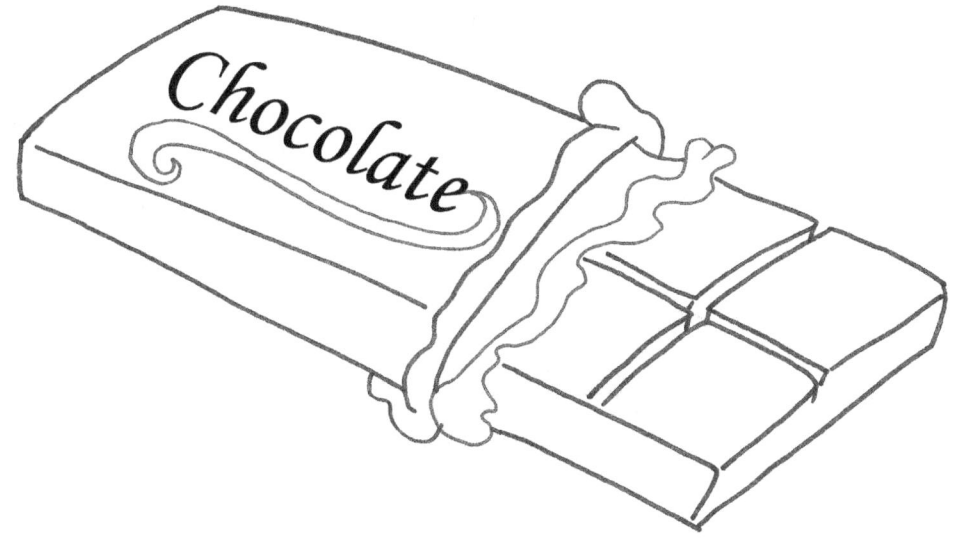

Avoid eating too much chocolate!

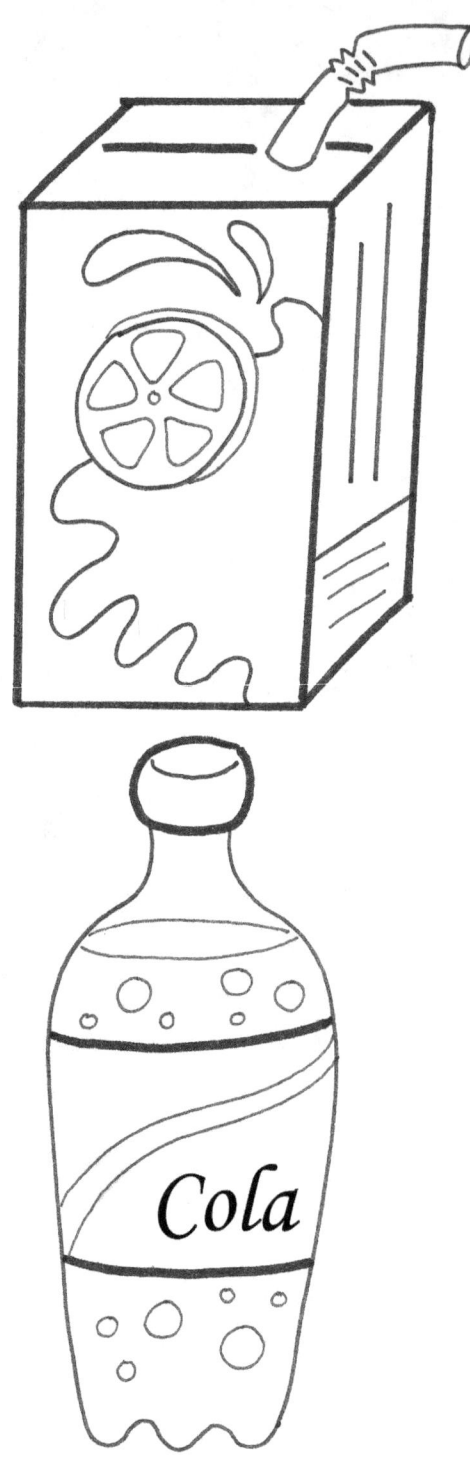

Avoid drinking sugary drinks like juice and carbonated drinks like soda.

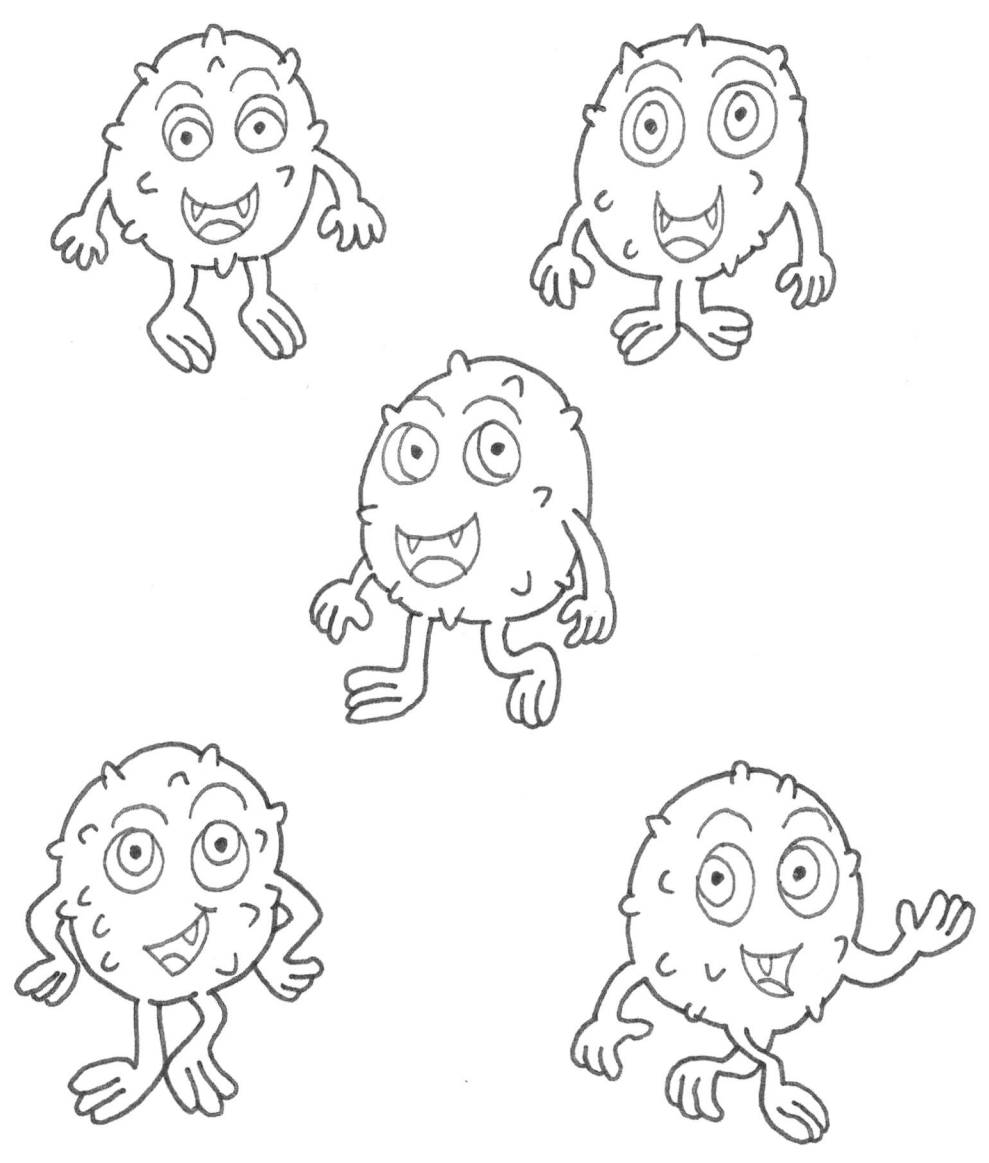

Hi there, we forgot to introduce ourselves!
Do you know who we are?

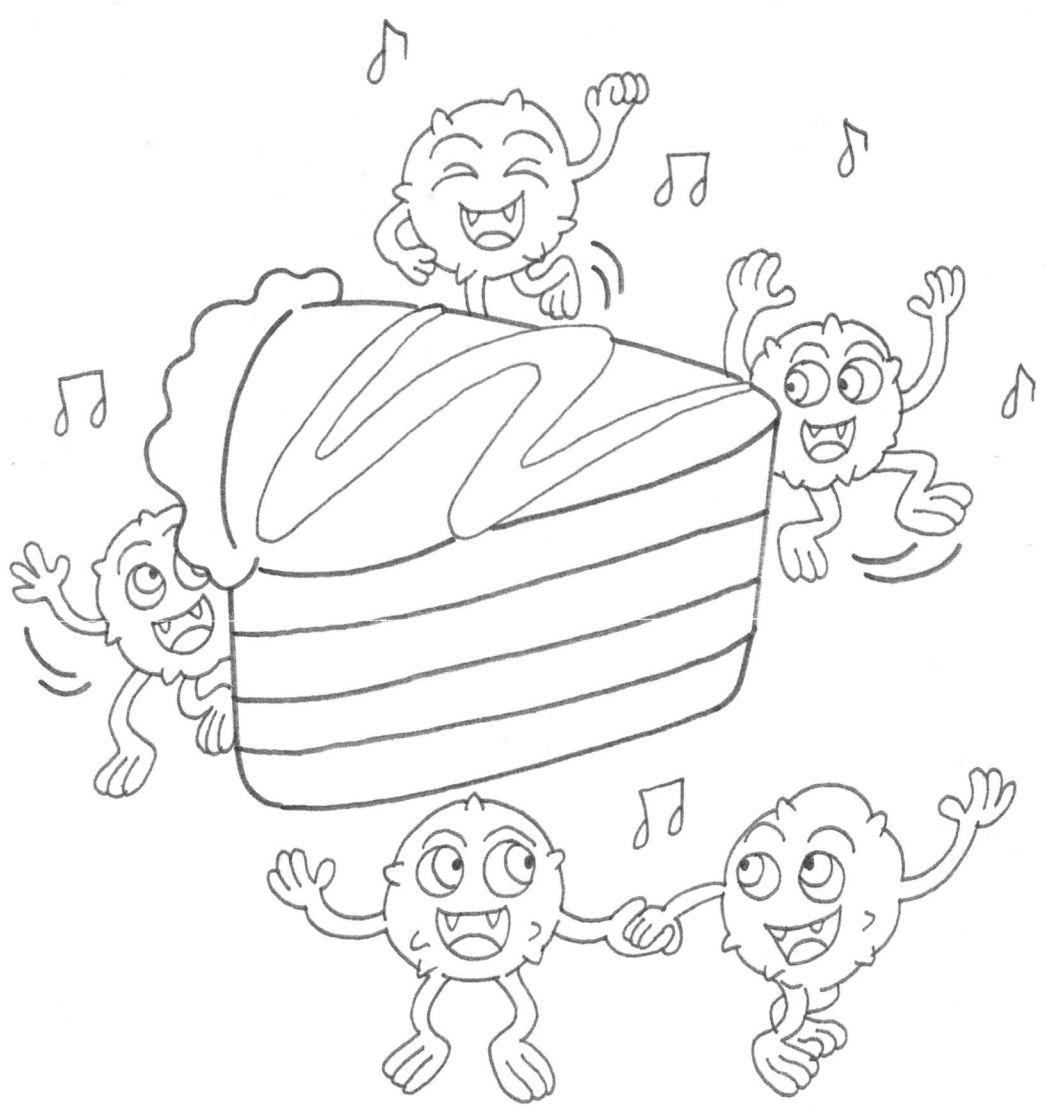

We are bacteria and we start to get very active and happy if you do not brush your teeth and if you eat a lot of sweets.

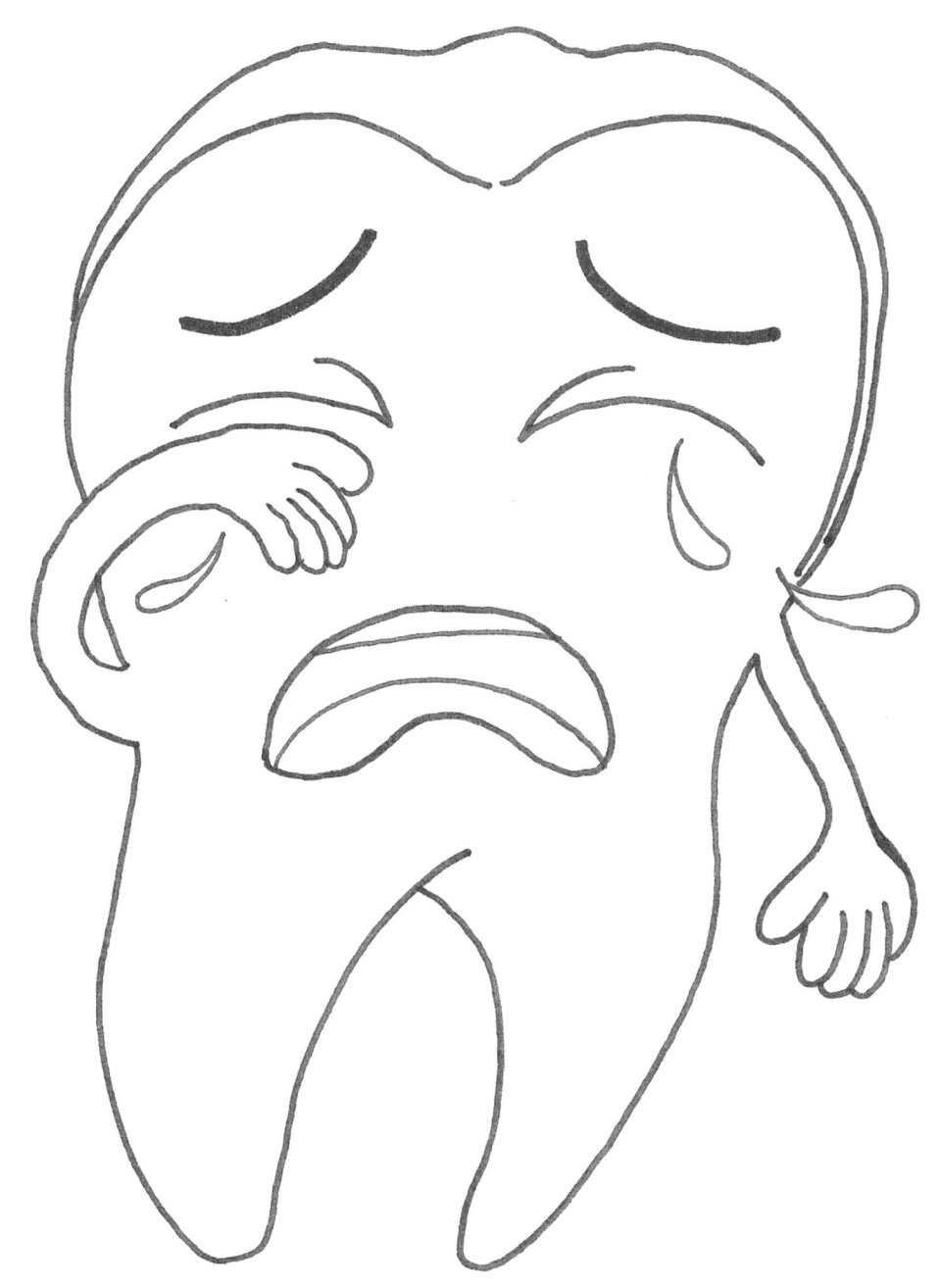

Food residue around your teeth, together with bacteria, will make your tooth sick if you do not brush your teeth properly.

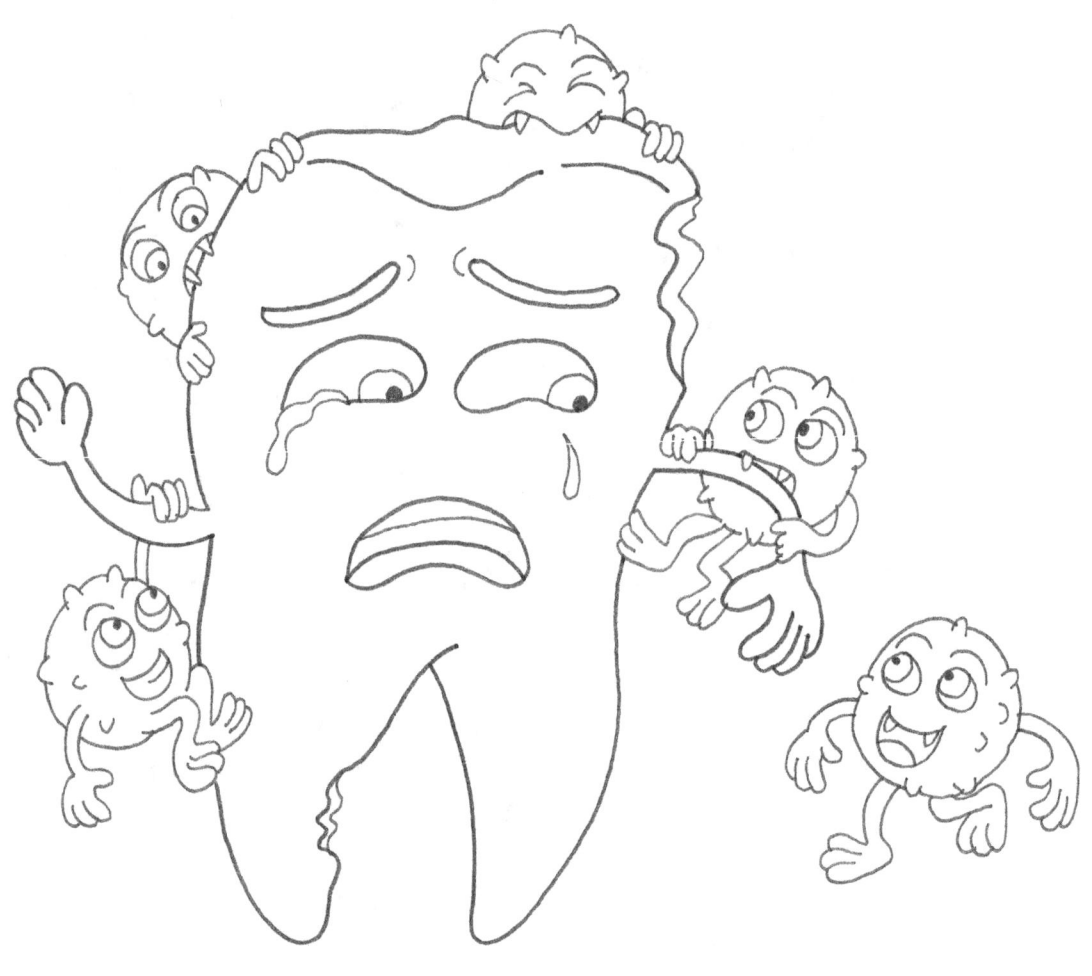

Party for bacteria but pain for you!

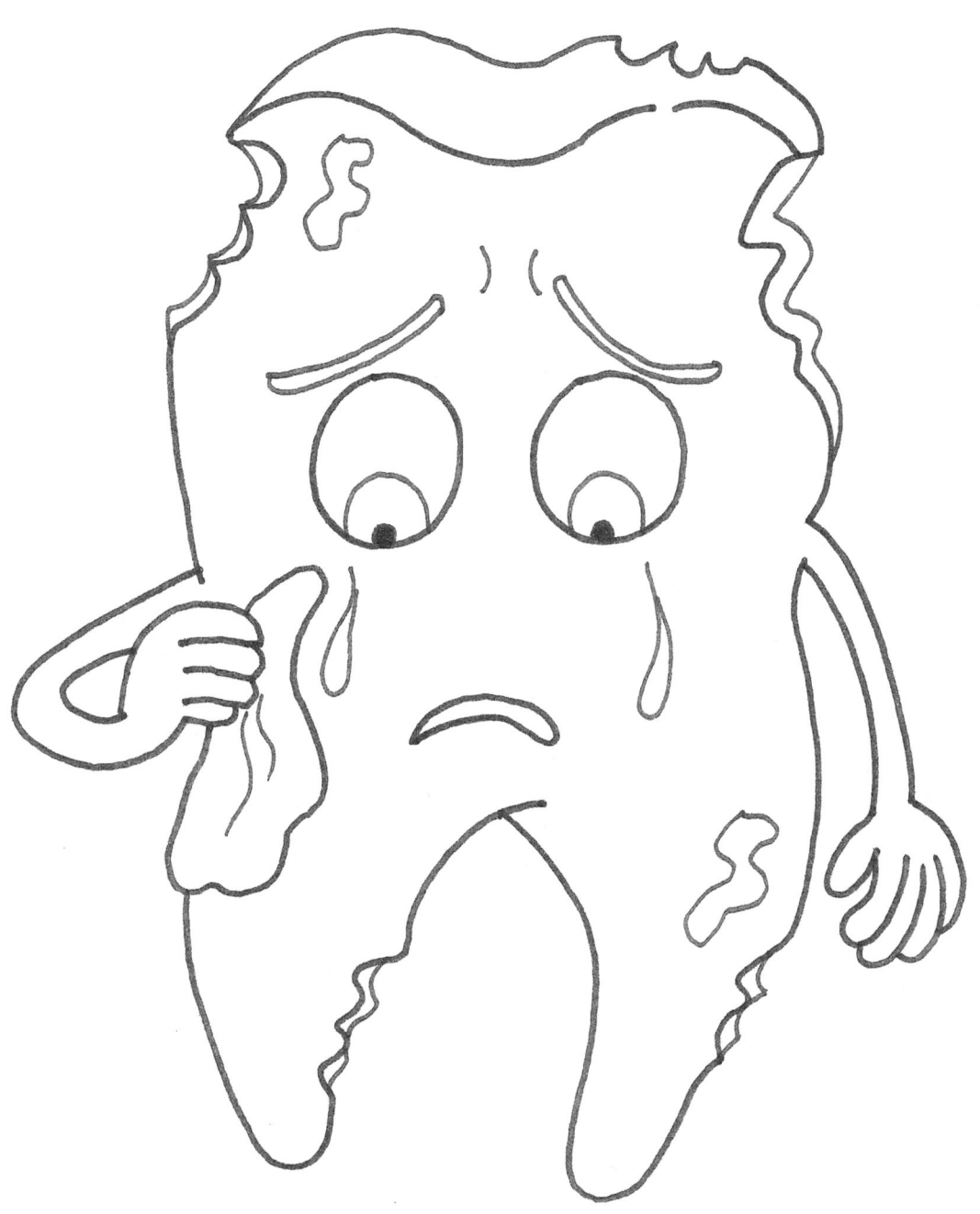

When a tooth is sick that means that you have tooth caries or tooth decay.

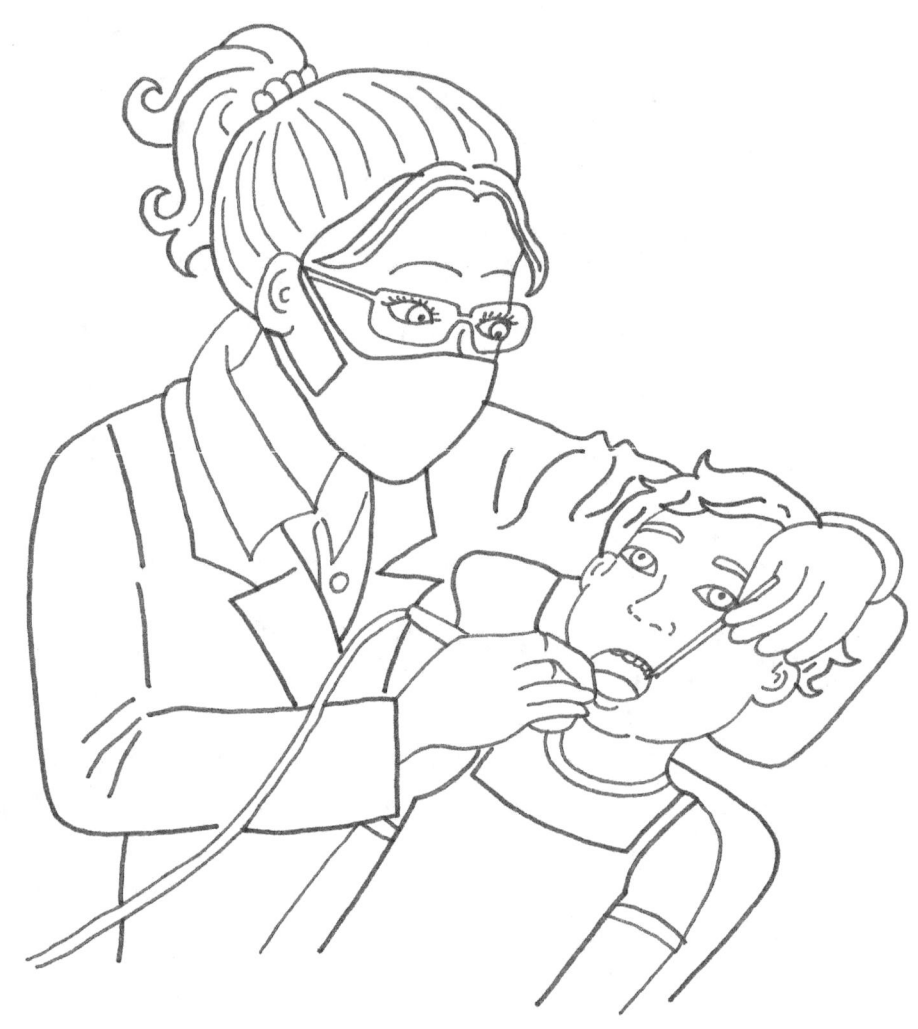

When that happens you have to visit your dentist.

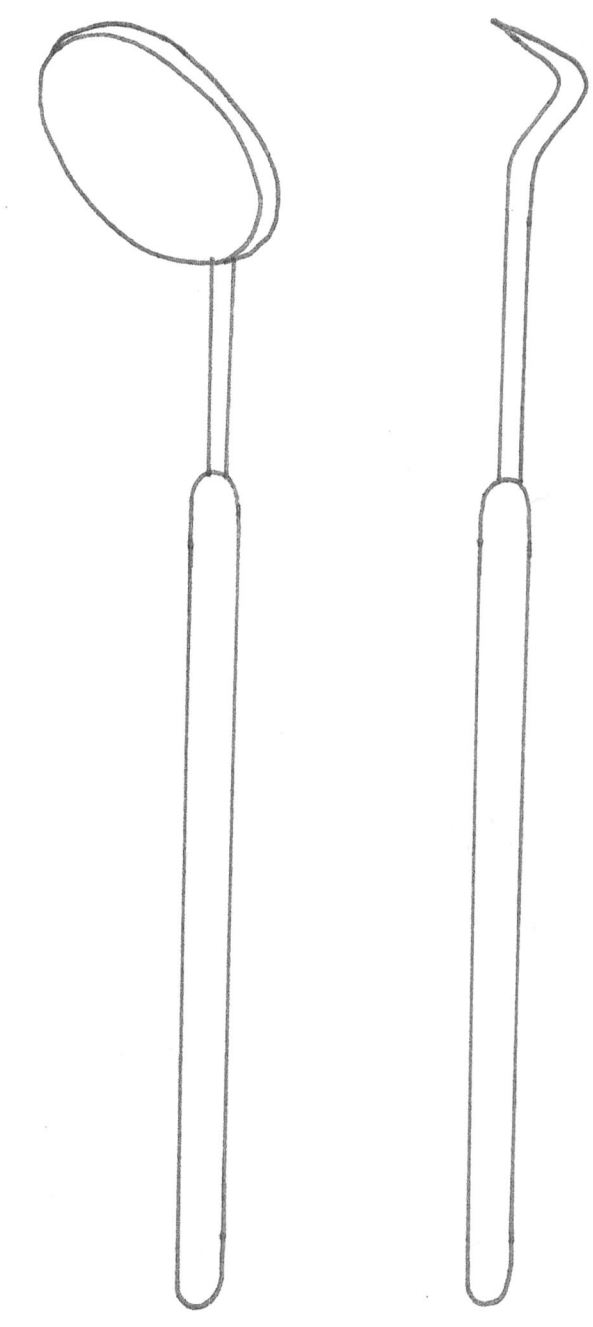

The dentist will use special tools to examine your teeth: mirror and explorer.

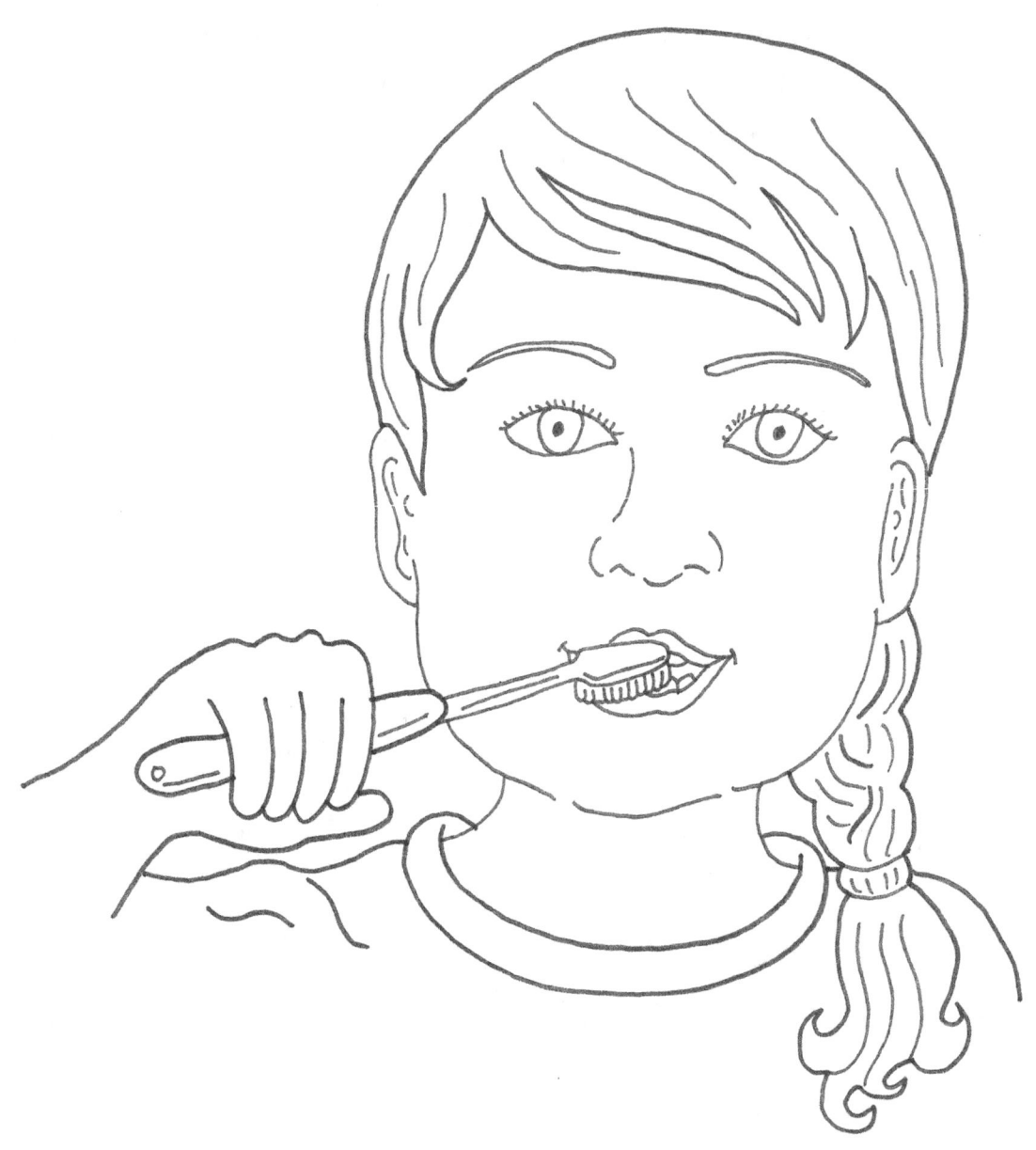

In order to make your teeth healthy you have to brush them at least twice a day.

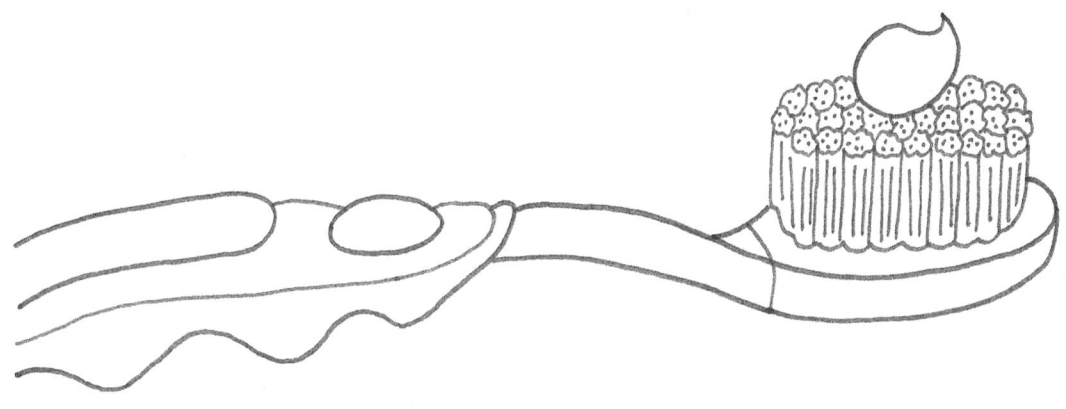

Put a pea size of paste or even less on a dry toothbrush...

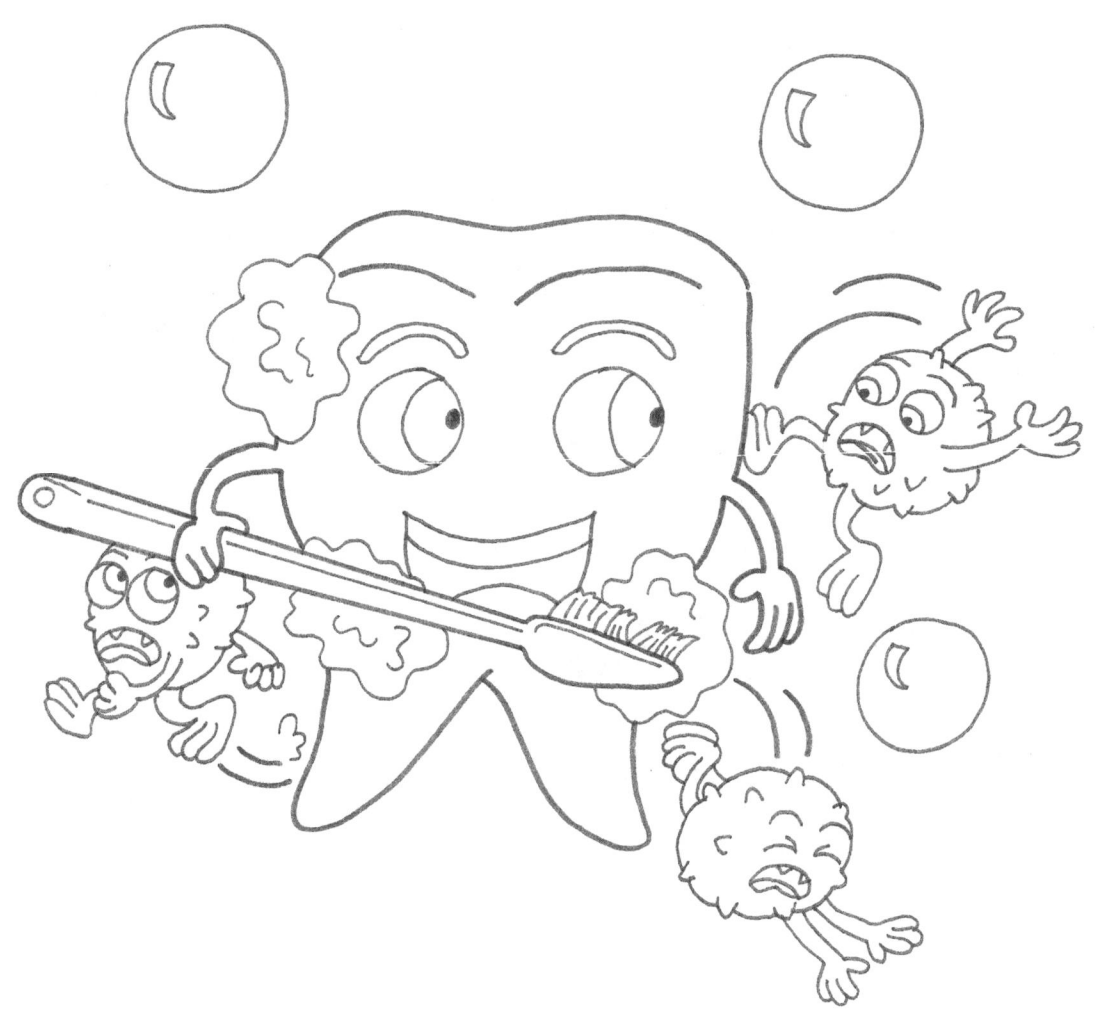

... and brush, brush, brush each tooth very carefully. ...

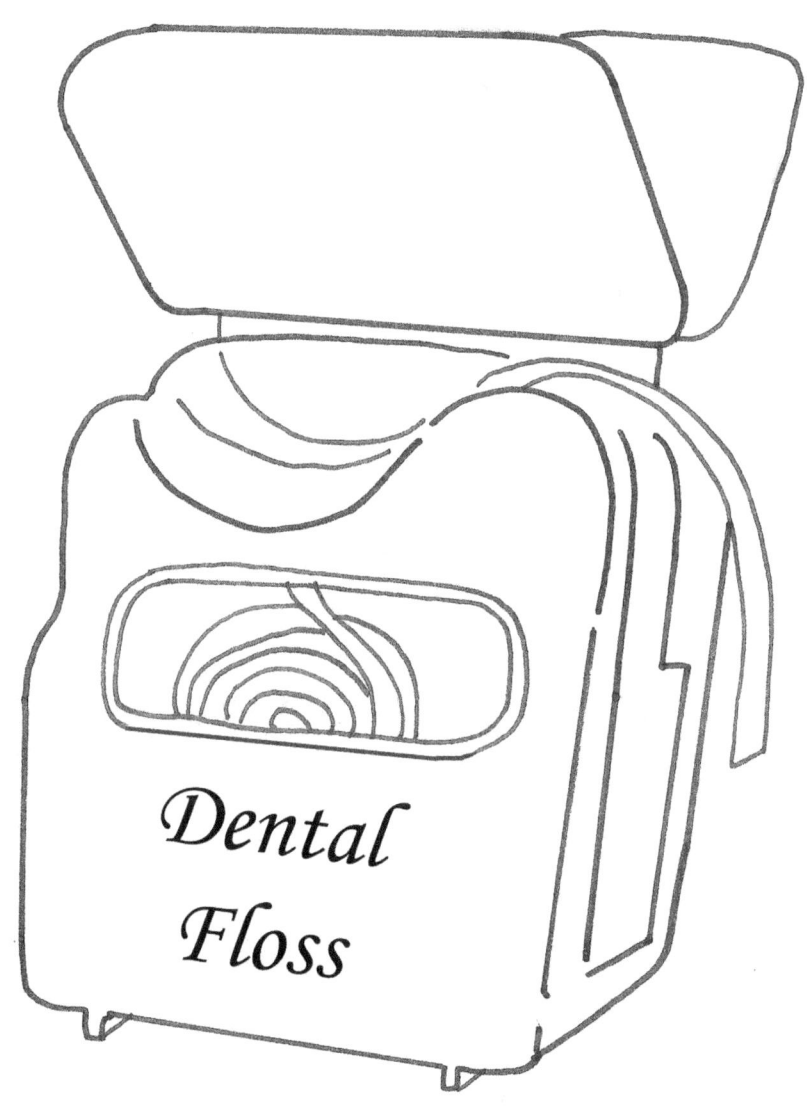

Do not forgot to floss!

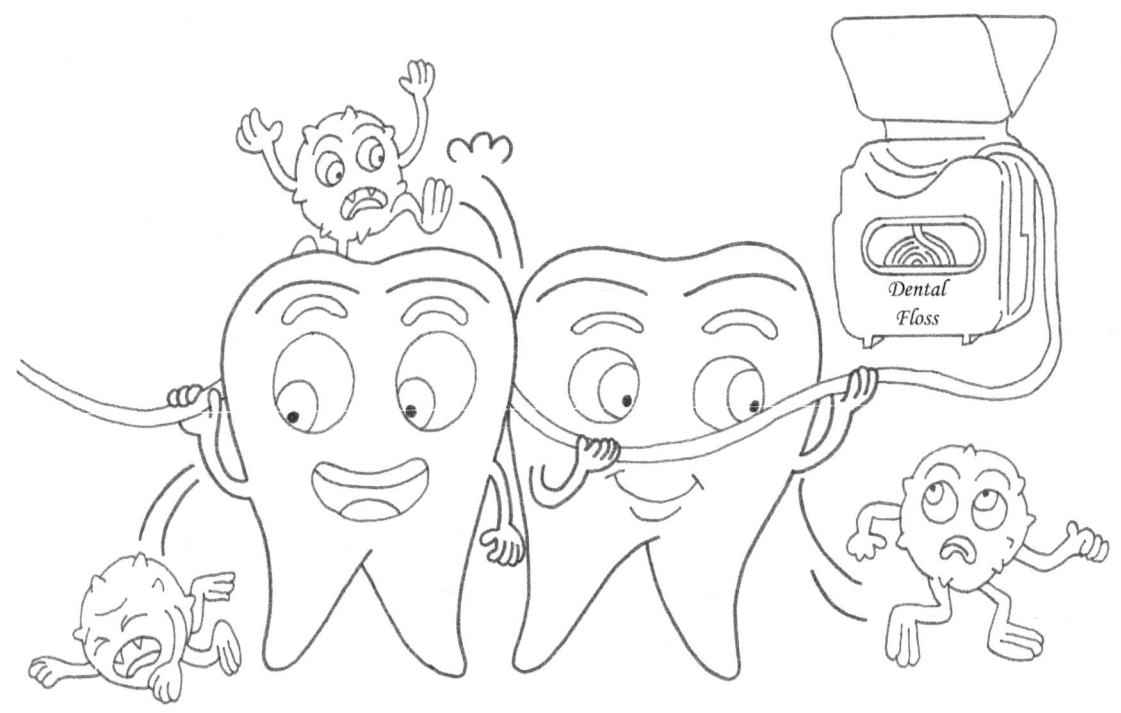

Floss between each tooth!

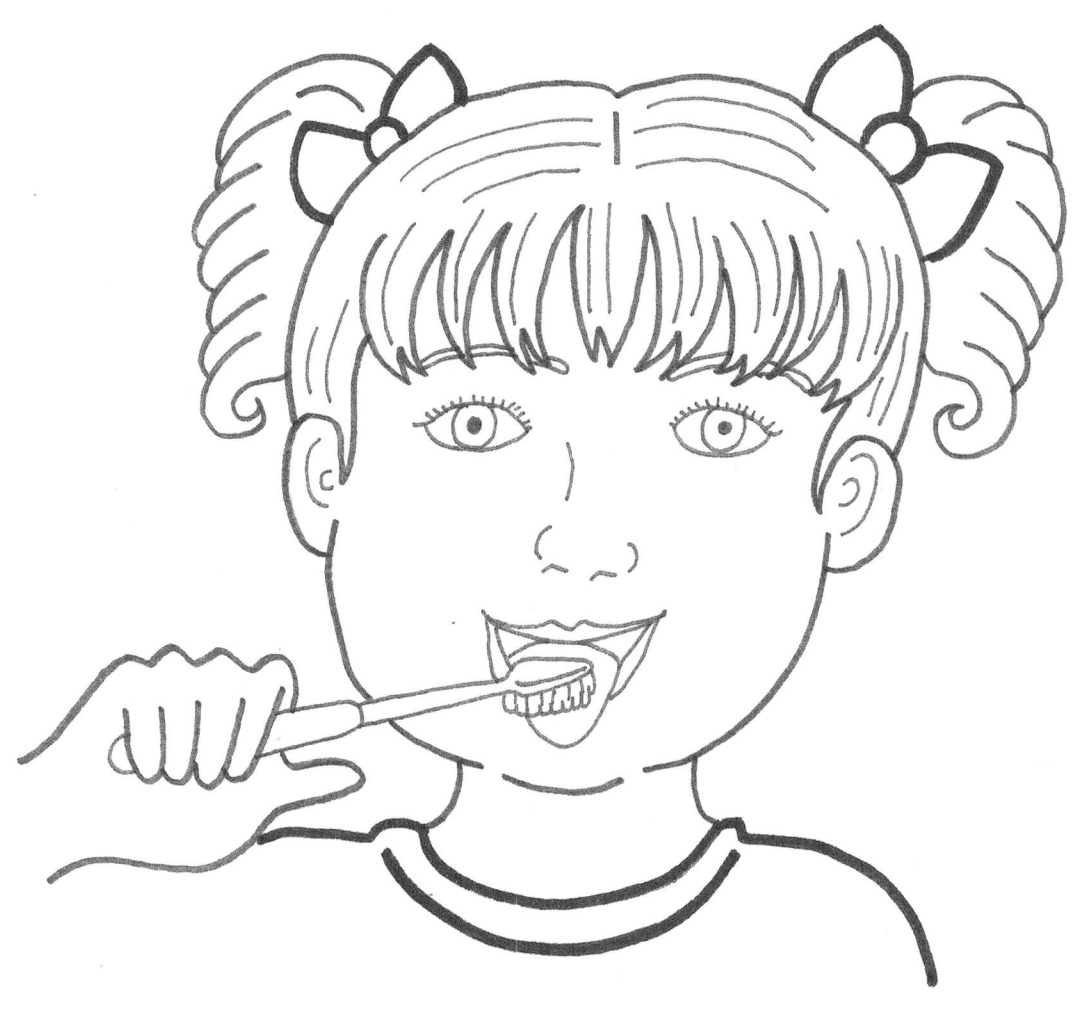

And do not forgot to clean your tongue as well.

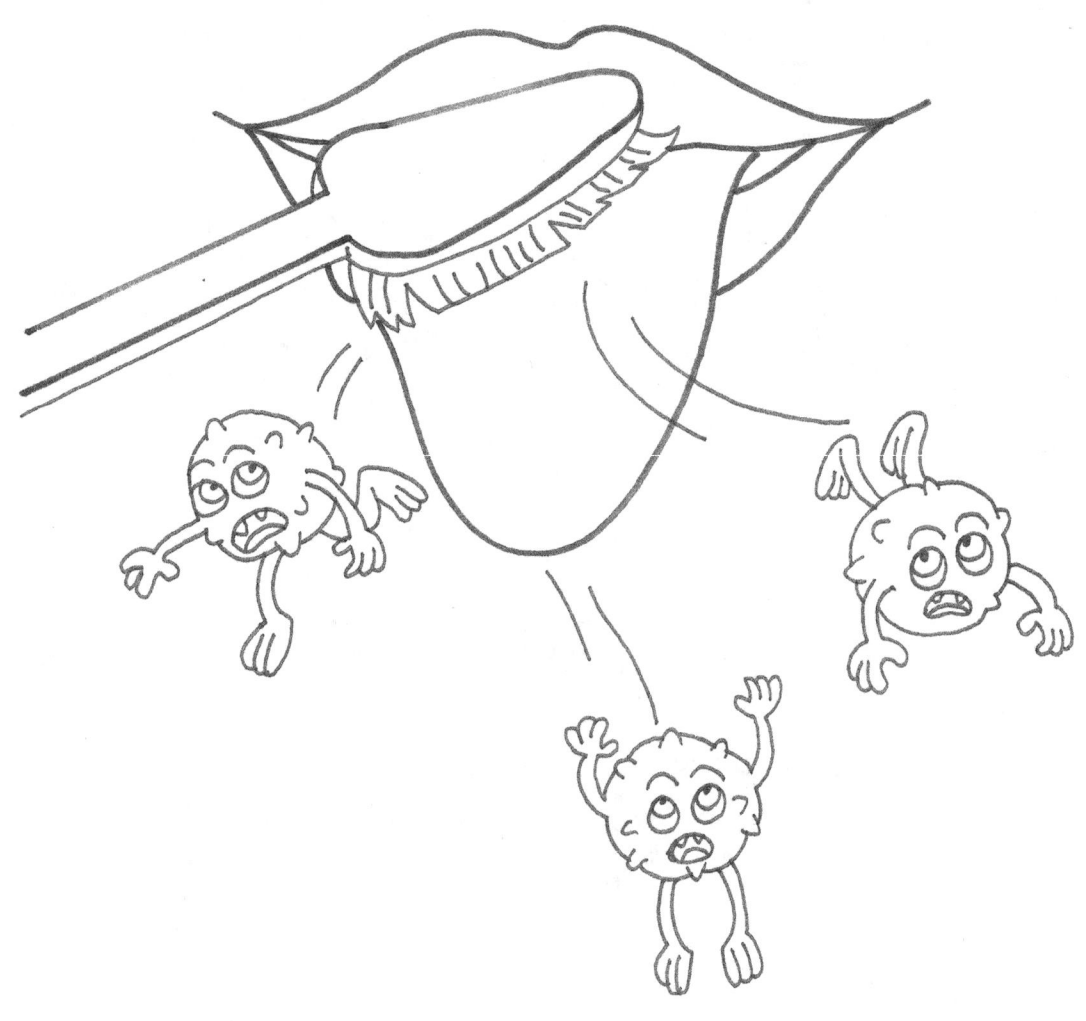

Brush the tongue gently with the toothbrush.

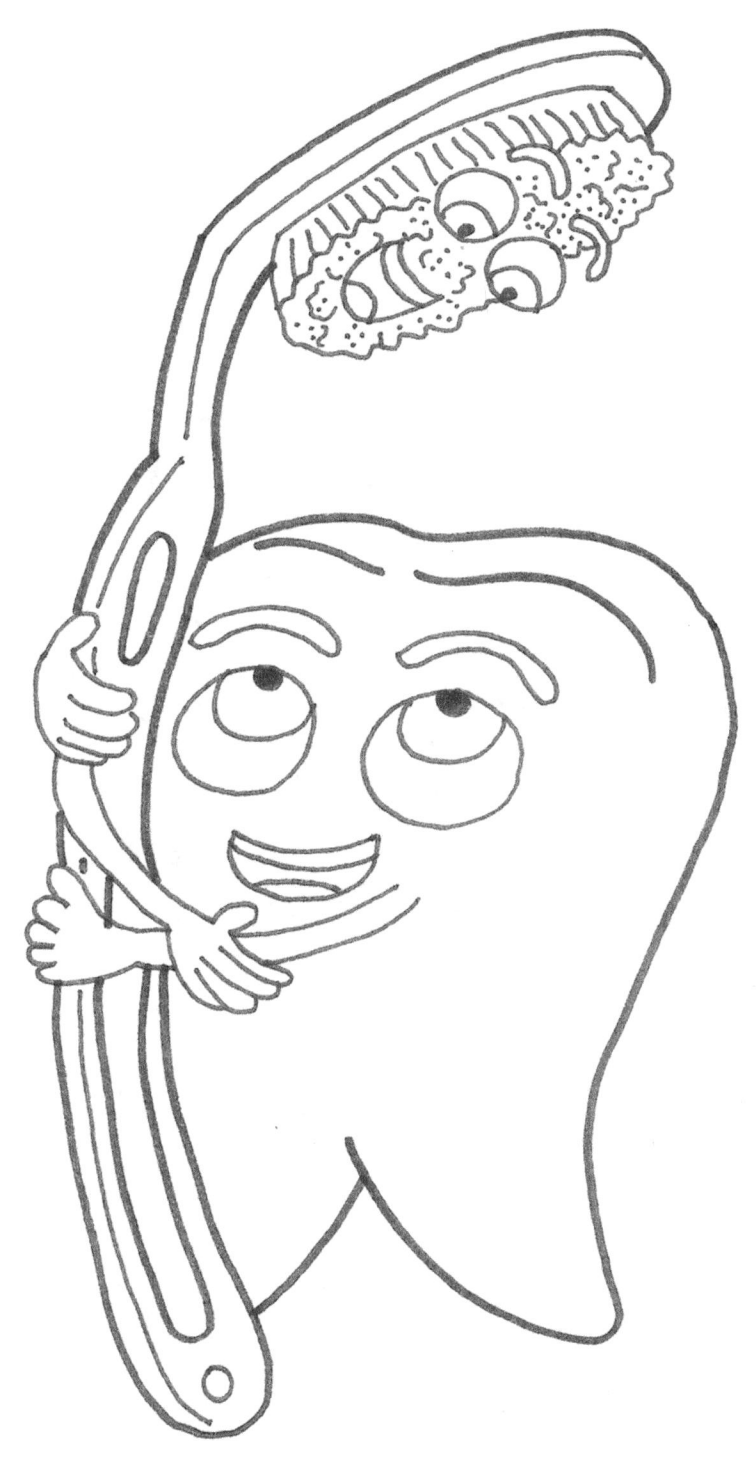

Love your toothbrush!

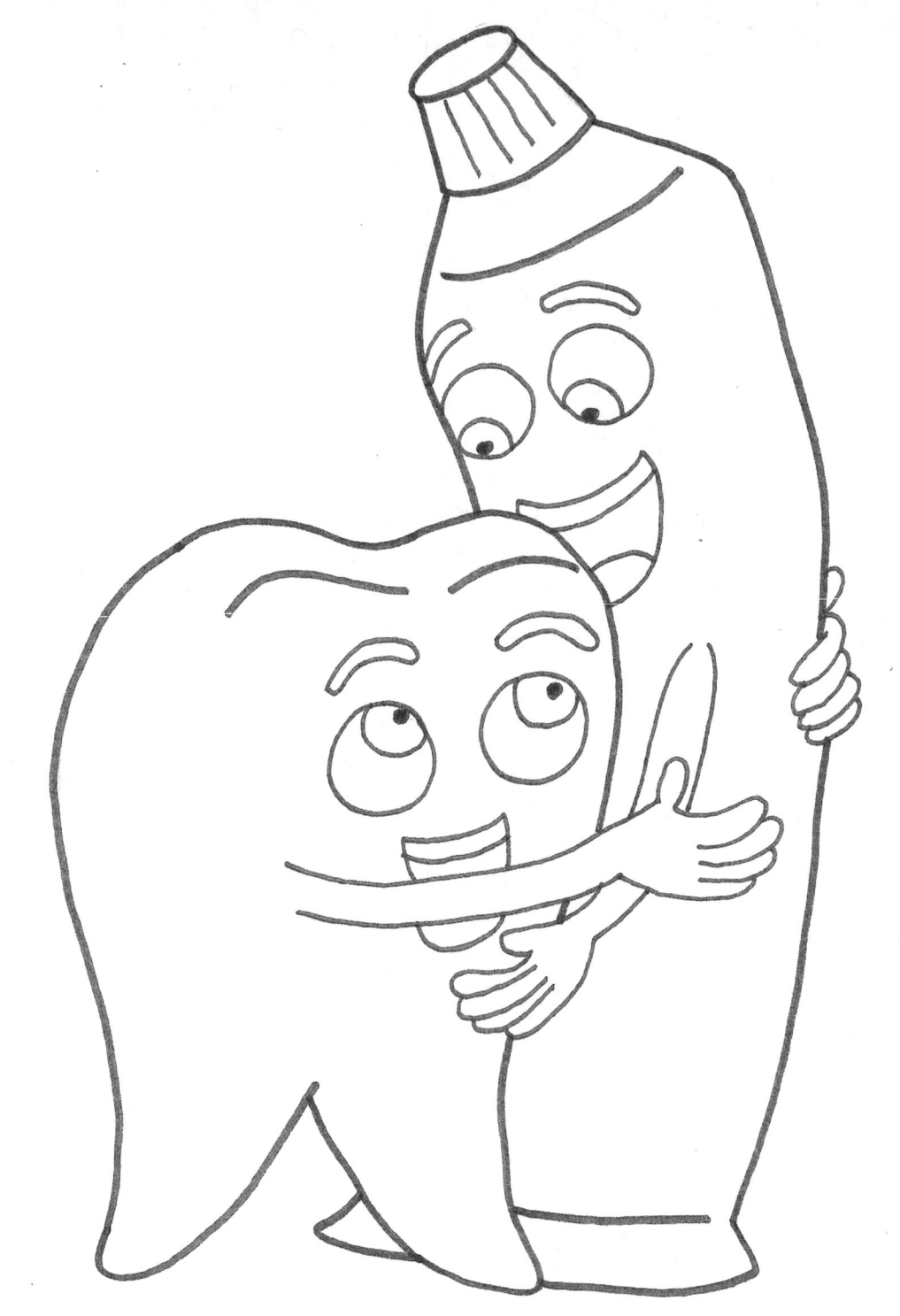

Love your toothpaste!

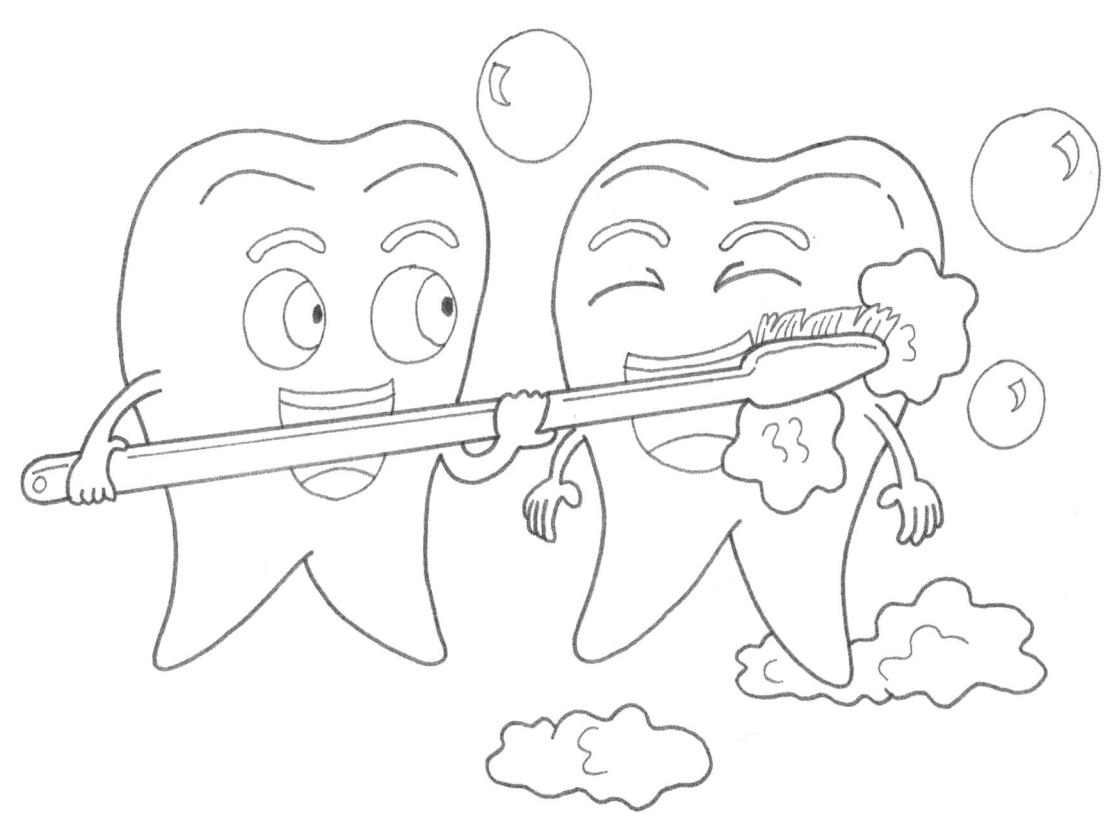

Lots of fun while brushing us!

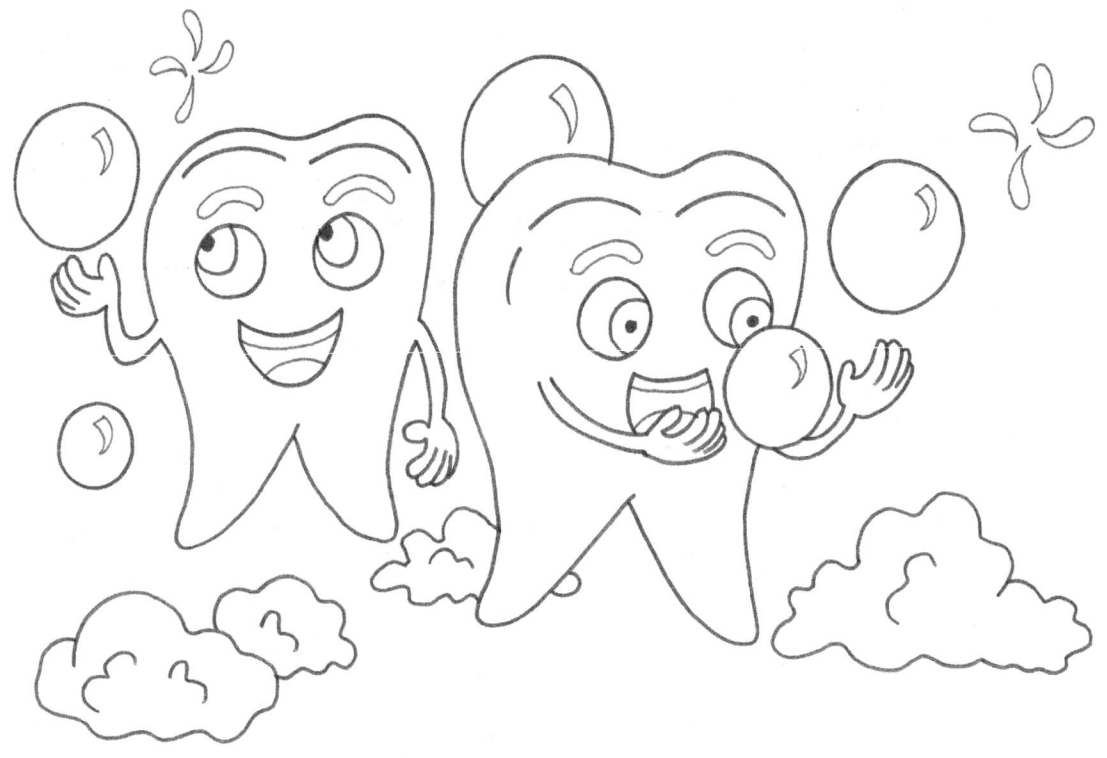

That makes us clean, healthy and happy!

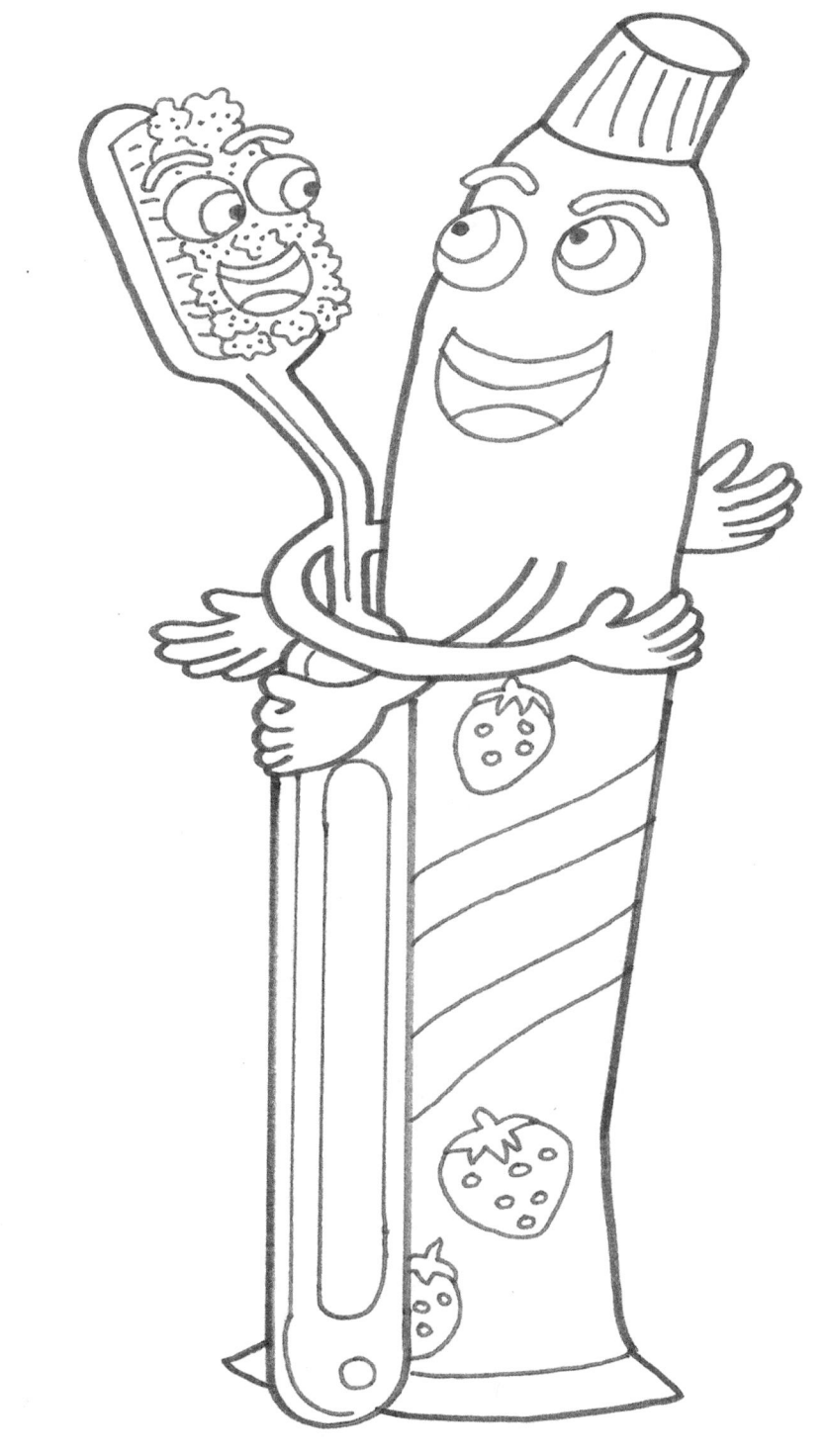

So what do you say?
You can do a great job with our help!

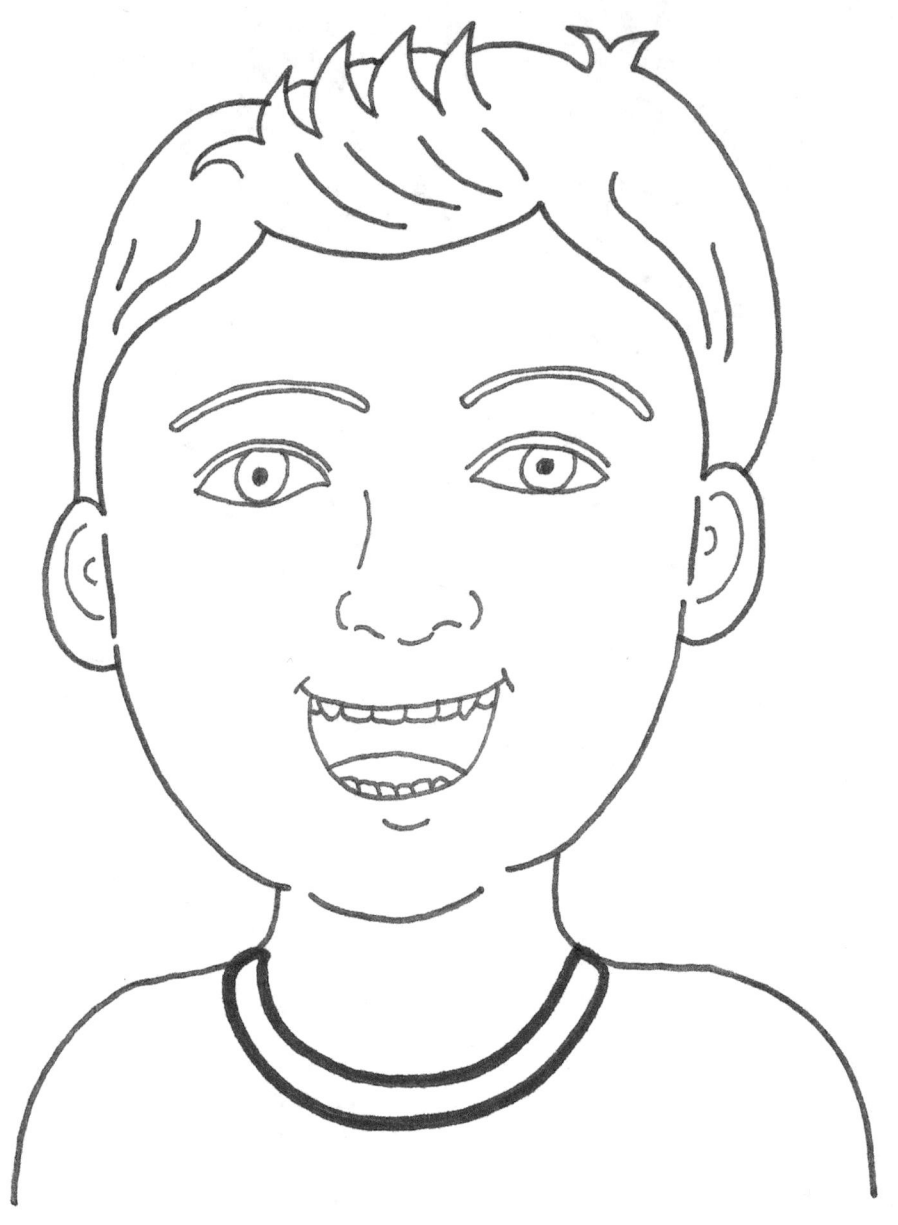

Just continue to keep your teeth clean and show to everyone your happy and beautiful smile!

www.ingramcontent.com/pod-product-compliance
Lightning Source LLC
Chambersburg PA
CBHW062206220526
45470CB00009B/2948